LOSING WEIGHT WITHOUT SPORTS AND DIETING

GET SLIM WITHOUT TORTURING YOURSELF WITH SPORTS AND DIETS --- TWELVE EASY STEPS TO YOUR DREAM WEIGHT

DAN HILD

ISBN 978-1-63940-692-0

Contents

Preface

Dear reader,

I want to thank you for your interest in my book! The fact that you are holding it in your hands is evidence that overweight is an important topic for you or a person close to you. It was the same for me!

People with „too much meat on their bones" often have to listen to advice like: „Eat half" or „do some sport". You and I know: It's not that easy. Overweight has various reasons, and the idea of being seen by others while doing sports is what makes most people avoid it. The chances of getting bombarded with appropriate or inappropriate commentary are just too high.

For many people suffering from obesity, doing sport is a horrific idea – and not because we are lazy or inactive. Many of us simply fear getting hurt. And diets have disappointed us time and time again. We just don't believe in it anymore. In the end we just torture ourselves for months, just to end up more obese than ever two or three months later.

In this book, I have compiled twelve simple approaches that will help you lose weight without heavy dieting or sports.

If you follow these approaches for some time, you will reach your personal dream weight, depending on your initial and desired weight.

I hope you have lots of success with that.

Sincerely, Dan Hill

ONE

Low Carb – Eating Few Carbohydrates

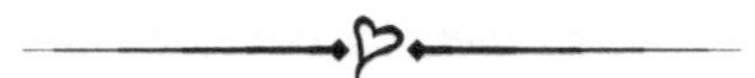

Have you heard of „satiating ingredients"? Some time ago, when meat was a rarity in daily meals, they included satiating ingredients instead. Those were important, as many people had to do hard physical work. Satiating ingredients could consist of potatoes, rice, pasta products, or simply bread.

Nowadays, most people live in other circumstances. Many work at a desk or do other physically not very demanding tasks. A „satiating ingredient" is pure poison for people with such a lifestyle. They supply their body with energy it doesn't need, and consequently stores away for a lack of alternatives.

That's why it makes sense to avoid carbohydrates as far as possible. That includes bread, pasta, pizza, potatoes, and everything containing sugar. For a change these things might be tasty. But in large quantities it is responsible for overweight. Scientific research has long proven that an overt consumption of carbohydrates has connections to cancer, multiple sclerosis, Alzheimer's, and diabetes. Dr. med. Ulrich Strunz has written a book on the topic, titled „Warum macht die Nudel dumm?".

If you want to lose weight, you should know that the body can gain energy much easier from carbohydrates than from fats. As long as the body has carbohydrates at its disposal, it will not burn fat, and it will surely not start using the fat depots it has stored away.

However, you should not only avoid the obvious carbohydrate sources, but also the hidden carbohydrate bombs. We all know that pasta and pastry contains loads of these ingredients, be that bread, croissants or crispbread. The classic sweets, as well as potatoes, are known to us as rich in carbohydrates. But we can also find hidden carbohydrates in the form of sugar in beverages (sweet drinks, wine, beer, alcohol) as well as in several processed foods. In the end, many of them contain sugar and forms of sugar like glucose, fructose and dextrose (grape sugar). Avoid all products containing these ingredients, and prepare your meals with fresh ingredients. If you do that, you know what you're eating. And with processed foods, get used to reading the product information.

TWO

GREEN TEA

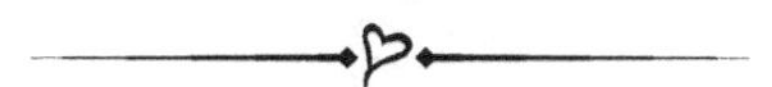

The beneficial effects of green tea (without sugar) have long been known in Asia. The caffeine contained drives the metabolism and with it the burning of fat in your body (calories as well).

Studies by the Tokyo-based „Health Care Products Research Laboratory" have shown that so-called catechins in green tea prevent the storage of fat in the liver and other tissues in mice. And the „American Journal of Clinical Nutrition" published a study on fat burning in which they prove that a frequent and appropriate consumption of catechins will result in sustainable fat burning.

Drunk in appropriate volumes, green tea is a healthy drink. If you want to lose weight, however, you should drink it unsweetened.

THREE
MAGNESIUM

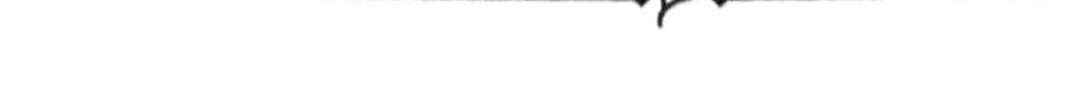

Magnesium plays an important role in burning fat. As enzyme building blocks and muscle minerals, the body needs magnesium in large quantities. Only with magnesium the body can burn fat efficiently.

Many experts are convinced that the bad balance of most diets can be attributed to a lack in magnesium. Thanks to the dietary restrictions, the body takes in even less magnesium than otherwise – and most people don't consume enough magnesium as it is. This has mostly to do with the fact that numerous foods drastically accelerate the magnesium breakdown. Especially Cola (and other lemonades as well) virtually flood out the magnesium – with consequences. Additionally the body needs more magnesium in times of stress or during sickness.

Different sources recommend various consumption volumes. I myself took in 200 milligrams extra in the morning and the evening each for a long time. By now, however, I take in twice that, and I feel awesome.

If there is a lack in magnesium, the body reduces the fat-burning. You start feeling tired and exhausted. Signs of magnesium deficiency can be cramps in the legs, but they can also include sleeping problems.

FOUR

CHILI

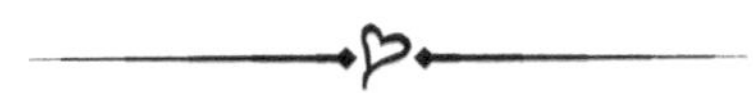

Chili is known as a hot spice. Some kinds of chili are so hot that eating them can actually be unhealthy for some people. Responsible for that is the alkaloid capsaicine within the spice.

This ingredient leads to the organism heating up. Experts call that thermogenesis. This is also used by experts, however, to create chili-based agents for fighting pain.

Thermogenesis is a process in which the organism quickly turns energy into heat. And if your diet is low in carbs and fats, using the fat storages is the most sensible point of attack. In this case, the chili is a real fat-burner. Additionally, chili consumption raises the temperature. The body reacts with sweating in order to cool down, which uses up additional energy.

Also chili has antibacterial and anti-inflammatory effects and promotes the production of bile acid, which supports the digestion and the burning of fat.

One main ingredient of the chili pepper, DHC, has been studied thoroughly in various American research papers. The test subjects ingested a capsule of DHC on a daily basis for a longer period of time. It became apparent that the test subjects burned twice as much fat as the comparison group who only received a placebo.

Despite these marvellous characteristics, you should not consume too many (and too hot) chilli peppers, as they can harm the oral mucosa and the stomach.

FIVE

GINGER

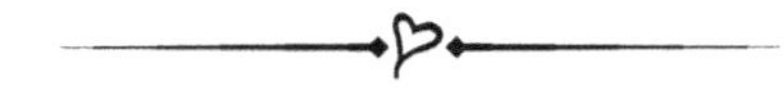

Similar to chilli peppers, ginger supports the metabolism and the heat-production. Furthermore the lemon-yellow root promotes the production of bile acid, which in turn drives the burning of fat and makes sure that heavy food is digested more easily.

Ginger can even be cultivated in our latitudes. Just put a root in some earth.

Furthermore, the ginger root contains a large number of anti-oxidants. These bind free radicals, preventing various diseases.

The root also contains lots of vitamin c and calcium, magnesium, iron, potassium, sodium and phosphorus. It is an amazing source of micronutrients.

SIX
PROTEINS

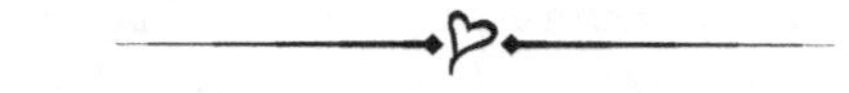

Protein is a central factor for sustainable weight reduction. During my diets I kept noticing again and again that muscle mass and water were the first to go. Depending on the water percentage of the diet, its reduction can be positive or negative. A reduction of muscle mass, however, is always negative.

Muscles are the most important burning mechanism for calories. Even during the night, every muscle cell burns energy: 24 hours a day, seven days a week. If we lose muscle mass during a diet, it's as though you'd take one wing off a plane in order to have a lower take-off weight and fly better.

If we want to sustainably lose weight, and make our lives easier even after the diet, we should take in enough protein. Experts recommend 1.5 to 2.5 grams of pure protein per kilogram of body weight and day. That means that if you weigh 100 kilograms, you should take in 150 to 250 grams of protein per day.

Actually the body requires more energy to digest proteins than the proteins themselves deliver. Furthermore taking in protein-rich foods leads to a feeling of fullness much more quickly.

Of course you can take in proteins during your normal diet. Fish, meat, or dairy products are wonderful sources of protein. Vegetarians and vegans would use other products like tofu. Even some fruits and vegetables contain large quantities of protein. Note, though, that foods always contain calories and other ingredients. You will hardly lose weight if you take in your proteins through whole milk. One litre of whole milk contains roughly 33 grams of protein – at a body weight of 100 kilograms, that would mean a „milk demand" of 4.5 litres a day, equalling more than 3240 calories. Even with a light milk with 0.3 percent of fat, you would still take in 1800 calories extra – about the daily calorie demand of an adult.

More and more manufacturers start offering functional food containing large amounts of protein or protein-substitutes. There's nothing that would speak against that. Fact is, however, that many manufacturers not only add proteins to these foods, but also large quantities of sugars of all kinds (carbohydrates), and even preservatives. Read the information in the chapter „avoid additives".

Another possibility is using protein compounds used in sports diets. Many of these products contain high-quality whey protein. If you don't meet your protein demand through normal food and beverages, you can do it with these products. They, too, contain calories and various additives though.

Such drinks are made for people who do lots of sports and consequently use a lot of energy (calories). That means that you have to keep an eye on the calories and additives contained in the product of your choice. High amounts of sugar and artificial sweeteners like aspartame_are no rarity. Taking a good look will pay off.

[1]The Centre of Health writes on its website: „Aspartame, the sweetener with many side-effects, isn't half as harmless as studies provided by the manufacturers

claim. During its metabolisation it releases harmful neural toxins. Loss of memory, depression, blindness and loss of hearing are just some of its effects on the human organism." (http://www.zentrum-der-gesundheit.de/ia-aspartam-suessstoff.html)

SEVEN
LEMONS

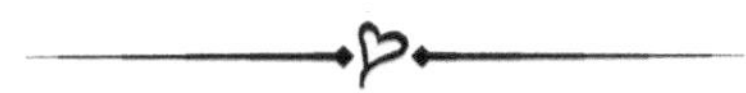

One of the most effective plants for losing weight is the lemon. It is surprising that it's not used in more dietary programs. This fruit has a lot to offer.

Drink the freshly pressed juice of two lemons each day. This supports the fat-burning in your body significantly. Or eat two lemons in order to also use the valuable pulp.

The juice can be diluted in water – just make your own lemonade! You should not sweeten it, however. And if you have to, do it with Stevia.

The lemon will help you in several ways:

- the digestion is improved
- the metabolism is supported (and with it the burning of calories)
- the blood pressure is optimised
- the cholesterol level is reduced
- the immune system is improved
- the blood vessels become more flexible

Additionally there is research that suggests lemons prevent the growth of cancer cells. Also these fruits are rich in vitamin c. This vitamin is used by our body for over 300 processes. Popular experts have recommended, during the last few years, to increase the intake of vitamin c significantly in order to prevent various illnesses.

If you eat lemons over the course of several days, you will soon notice that your body gets used to it, and the fruits no longer seem that sour to you.

The lemon is, by the way, metabolised basically, which is good news for people suffering from hyper-acidity.

EIGHT

GREEN COFFEE

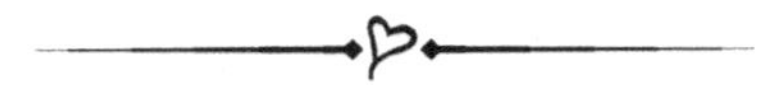

Green coffee, that is, unroasted coffee beans, have a high amount of caffeine. This drives the metabolism and with it the fat-burning processes. At the same time it contains a lot of hydrochloric acid. Based on this there are various products with green coffee extract being offered in stores. In my opinion, the author Peter Carl Simons is right when he states in his work[1] that instead of drinking the often very expensive extract, one can simply drink green coffee.

Hydrochloric acid is an important substance for supporting the fat reduction. Additionally it prevents the body from taking in sugars and fats. By roasting the coffee, however, it is destroyed to a large part, which is why there is hardly any of it left in „normal coffee".

Some research results showed evidence that green coffee also positively influences the blood sugar levels. And one study from the University of Scranton from 2012 confirms that people who drink green coffee can lose 10 percent of their weight even without changing anything else about their diet. Further research yielded similarly impressive results.

Green coffee can be enjoyed as an alternative to common coffee in the same amount.

[1]Simons, Peter Carl: Green Coffee - A weight loss guarantee? - How you can lose weight quickly and easily with green coffee, CreateSpace 2015

.

NINE

AVOIDING ADDITIVES

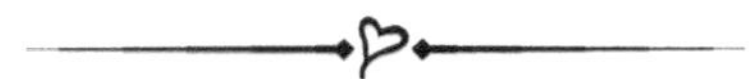

Do you know foods of which the manufacturers claim that they are lactose free, gluten free, contain no artificial sweeteners or no fat? Many internationally industrial food producers draw in customers with such claims. Meanwhile it is said that according labels have been created.

Basically there's nothing that would speak against a manufacturer highlighting certain ingredients of a product. He is even obligated to list all ingredients by law. But if they are printed on the packaging in large letters, you should keep in mind the following:

If a product is „lactose free" or „gluten free", it doesn't necessarily mean it's healthy – the opposite may even be the case! „Without added sugar" doesn't mean there's no sugar in it, but simply that there wasn't any sugar added. And it surely doesn't say anything about the value of the product for your health. Even „fat free" doesn't always mean healthy.

All advertising prints give reason to stay alert. Lactose and gluten are often replaced with other substances that we don't even want in our food. And in other cases, too, it is sensible to read up on what the manufacturers bring to your plate. When in doubt, keep to fresh and natural foods.

TEN

DRINK WATER

Probably the simplest method for losing weight is replacing all your beverages with water. Be that the coffee for breakfast, the hot chocolate, the energy drink, the soft drink, the beer, or the wine after work: All of them contain calories and most of them no little amount. Simply by avoiding these drinks, most people could reduce their calorie intake by up to 50 percent – and that will quickly become visible on the scale.

When I am talking about „water", I mean the liquid that the waterworks send through our pipes, and no carbonated mineral water. On one hand carbon dioxide is an acid. It literally acidifies our body, which can have negative effects on many organic processes that support the weight loss. Also, water from the tap is no worse than most expensive mineral waters in most areas.

If you're in doubt, just ask at your local waterworks. Most people, however, can stop hauling water bottles. At the same time you can prevent a lot of environmental harm created by the transport of bottles around half the globe. It is best to just drink the water you have at hand, which many people use for their coffee or tea anyway.

ELEVEN

SLEET YOURSELF SLIM

In 2004, the Clinical Research Center of the University of Chicago conducted research in which the night's rest of the test subjects was reduced. As little as two nights with four hours of sleep yielded dramatic results. The sleep deprivation increase the hunger by 24 percent, and the appetite by 23 percent. The test subjects especially craved sweet and salty foods with many carbohydrates and a high amount of calories.

The internationally renowned sleep researcher Prof. Eve Van Cauter prove that people suffering from sleep deprivation develop a ravenous appetite for carbohydrates like bread, pasta or sweets.

At the same time, these people are less willing to work during the day. As a result, they move less and use less energy (calories).

The results from these observations could be confirmed through blood analyses: People who slept less had a loss in the satiating hormone leptin by 18 percent, and an increase in the appetite-driving hormone ghrelin by 28 percent.

If you sleep frequently and long enough, you have a much lower risk of obesity in accordance with these research results. What you do with this information is up to you.

TWELVE

THINK YOURSELF SLIM

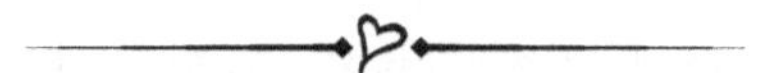

What are you thinking of yourself? Maybe you have heard that thinking affects the reality. And in reality, obese people especially have trouble imagining themselves as anything but „fat".

Commentary from the surroundings – party well-meant – show them again and again how others evaluate their body. After some time, many people give up. They feel like they lost to their own obesity and can't do anything about it. Henry Ford, the founder of the automotive corporation of the same name, said: „No matter if you think you can or can not do something, you are right."

You can not lose weight if you choose to „just try it". That has to do with your attitude. If you „try" something, you accept that you may not be successful – and that's what will happen. Only if you imagine that there is no alternative for losing weight, you will do just that: „Lose weight".

Furthermore, Henry Ford said: „There are more people who give up than those who fail." Indeed, many people are obese because they just give up. I don't want to exclude myself from those – I was the same.

Many people bringing a large number of kilos to the scale will also recognise this pattern in other areas of their life. They give up and think: „I can't do that anyway" or „I won't make it anyway". Or the worst: „I'll just give it a try".

Stop it! Don't think about the failure from the start! Don't think about the possibility of it „not working", but focus on reaching your goal.

Look forward to all the things you can do once you've scaled your peak. Imagine your new life! In fact it is very helpful to create pictures or collages about how your life will be at your dream weight. Indulge in your wildest dreams.

What will become of:

- Partnership / Love / Sexuality
- Family
- Friend circles
- professional situation
- acknowledgements from your surroundings
- physical well-being
- health
- luck
- …

Why should you not be able to do something thousands of other people could do despite being a lot heavier than you?

Understand me correctly: This task is not about escaping into a dream world. That would mean giving up again. It is about consciously knowing why you take the task of losing weight upon yourself. And every change in weight *is* stress and effort. From the reply to the why questions, you gain your motivation. The imagination what you will do once you leave the hard times behind you will help overcoming setbacks.

Imagine a top athlete. What results do you think a ski ace, a sprinter or a Formula 1 race driver would get if he went into the competition to „just try it"? Imagine Michael Schumacher's career, had he just started every race with the thought of „just making it through somehow". Winners are on the rostrum from the start. They feel the tingle of the champaign shower on their skin and the acknowledgements of the audience. If you don't feel that, want that, and are obsessed by it, you will never have it.

You have to motivate yourself the same way if you want to reach your desired weight. Be ready for hard tasks, and accept one or the other waiver. If you manage to motivate yourself, you will reach your desired weight, and surmount all obstacles in your way.

THIRTEEN
DO NOT HIDE

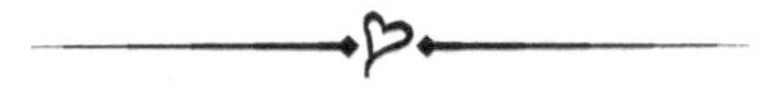

The book is titled „Losing weight without sports", and I want to keep this promise. We all know that doing sport in appropriate amounts is a good thing and helps keeping your body healthy. However, I will not recommend any exercises to you here.

What I want to recommend to you, however, is to not go the easiest way, and most importantly: not to hide.

A nice acquaintance of mine, Sonja, was told by many people from the start: „You are fat!", „You are ugly!", „Lose weight already!" and many more things obese people hear day after day. If you are exposed to such comments frequently, you try to avoid them. Sonja left her house more and more rarely, and even got her groceries delivered. She would have had more contact to the outside world if she had committed a crime and gone to prison.

Her life was limited to her small 50sqm apartment, where she lived and made money from home. When she wasn't working, she mostly sat in front of the TV looking at the world that she shut herself out of. Along with a lack of movement, she had increasing fear of „the world out there". Her loneliness, fear and sadness lead to her eating even more. Sonja gained weight.

As she also never went out to buy clothes, she ordered them from an American distributor for oversized clothing, or had pieces custom-made by online tailors.

As one day Sonja noticed heavy pain, she tried getting better herself in fear of going to the doctor, where people could disparagingly look down on her. Only when the pain became too unbearable, she consulted a doctor, who immediately sent her to the hospital. Along with the medical care she received psychological support that continued on after her hospital stay. The therapists helped her, so that nowadays she can leave the house again. Sometimes Sonja says that God sent her the pain to save her life. By now she has lost half of her overweight, and is working on losing the rest.

Today Sonja knows what she had done to herself when she decided to hide. If you are feeling a similar way, consult a coach or a nutritionist who can support you.

FOURTEEN
DAILY ACTIVITIES

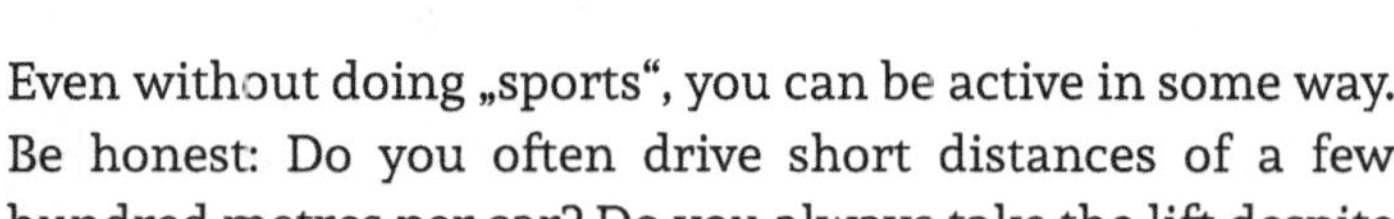

Even without doing „sports", you can be active in some way. Be honest: Do you often drive short distances of a few hundred metres per car? Do you always take the lift despite there being a staircase right next to it?

If you want to lose weight, you will have to change your relationship to your body step by step. Take the stairs once in a while, especially if it's just one or two floors. Leave your car in the driveway once in a while. Take some extra steps, or buy in stores that don't have a customer parking lot. In short: Try doing away with automatisms. Some people have gotten used to never moving if the movement can be done by a machine. Others reflexively grab their favourite beer from the fridge before setting the grocery bags down.

It is also very good to just take a walk for half an hour. Explore an area without any hassle, or go window-shopping – after the stores have closed, so there's less temptation. Find a hobby that gets you out of your house. Do you know geocaching? That's fun for the whole family, and you don't have to be particularly sporty (depending on the chosen destination). In the internet you can find lots of information about it. Or ask your neighbour if you can take their dog for a walk once in a while.

As I said, this is not about you suddenly becoming a top athlete. But you should start, step by step, to move your bones and muscles some more. And find out, what's fun for you.

FIFTEEN
SURGERY

More and more people choose to get under the knife in order to master their obesity through surgery. A short stay in the hospital seems like the easiest way to solve the problem.

But every surgery comes with risks, and for a person with significant overweight, the complications are much larger than for fit people. Many ignore that.

During our whole life we have heard that obese people live shorter lives anyway. Death by surgery, or larger physical damage, seems like a bearable risk. After the surgery we might have a normal weight so we can live a longer, healthier, and better life.

Unfortunately it is hard to find reliable figures for success and failure of surgery methods of this kind. It is a fact, however, that many people have paid for such measures with their health, or their lives. In many cases, the success was just temporary, and the obesity returned – similarly to diets – after a short time.

The Swiss diet coach Christoph Bisel, who looks after morbidly obese people in his office and also supports them online, reports his own experiences in his impressive book

„I was a beached whale“:

I started off the year 2014 at a weight of 320 pounds. Keep in mind that I had reached my maximum "fighting weight" more than a decade earlier, when I loaded my scale with a total of 350 pounds. What followed was the before mentioned surgeries. One of them in the year 2000 had a complication, which almost solved all my problems for good. The past years clearly brought along a tendency of increase.

I had lost part of my intestine due to a ruptured suture with subsequent peritonitis, which almost put an end to my "earthly suffering". At this point I have to confess that I have always loved my life and I am still loving it. Another side effect of the gastric bypass was a drastic weight loss which brought me down to somewhere around 140 pounds, mostly due to my feeble frame failing to ingest food. As soon as I had recovered from the effects of the surgery, my body gradually but persistently kept grabbing those lost pounds again. At the beginning of this year I realized that things could not go on that way. I certainly did not want to arrive back at the 350 pound mark! I believe I am an expert on all issues linked to being fat, including any you will ever read in any book, or experience, be it personally or among friends or acquaintances. In any case, it has surely been enough experience to know perfectly well how absolutely annoying it is to be living one`s life as a "beached whale". Some overweight people may deny that, just like I do, whenever something is at stake. But let`s be honest and agree upon the fact that the advantages of being fat are rather limited.

Meanwhile I now weigh less than 240 pounds. It has been more than 20 years since my scale last indicated that number. Does that mean I should still be considered a beached whale? Well, objectively speaking you may say this is a clear yes. My BMI (body mass index) is still located in a region that is commonly considered to be pathological. Whereas I feel downright slim when I think of all the way I have come in the endeavor to optimize my weight. After all it seems to be that overweight is a relative term.

I do not know your case, which is why I can't say whether or not an operation makes sense for you. What I can tell you, however: NEVER go into a surgery simply because it seems like the easiest way!

Disclaimer

Introduction

By using this book, you accept this disclaimer in full.

No advice

The book contains information. The information is not advice and should not be treated as such.

No representations or warranties

To the maximum extent permitted by applicable law and subject to section below, we exclude all representations, warranties, undertakings and guarantees relating to the book.

Without prejudice to the generality of the foregoing paragraph, we do not represent, warrant, undertake or guarantee:

- that the information in the book is correct, accurate, complete or non-misleading.

- that the use of the guidance in the book will lead to any particular outcome or result.

Limitations and exclusions of liability

The limitations and exclusions of liability set out in this section and elsewhere in this disclaimer: are subject to section 6 below; and govern all liabilities arising under the disclaimer or in relation to the book, including liabilities arising in contract, in tort (including negligence) and for breach of statutory duty.

We will not be liable to you in respect of any losses arising out of any event or events beyond our reasonable control.

We will not be liable to you in respect of any business losses, including without limitation loss of or damage to profits, income, revenue, use, production, anticipated savings, business, contracts, commercial opportunities or goodwill.

We will not be liable to you in respect of any loss or corruption of any data, database or software.

We will not be liable to you in respect of any special, indirect or consequential loss or damage.

Exceptions

Nothing in this disclaimer shall: limit or exclude our liability for death or personal injury resulting from negligence; limit or exclude our liability for fraud or fraudulent misrepresentation; limit any of our liabilities in any way that is not permitted under applicable law; or exclude any of our liabilities that may not be excluded under applicable law.

Severability

If a section of this disclaimer is determined by any court or other competent authority to be unlawful and/ or unenforceable, the other sections of this disclaimer continue in effect.

If any unlawful and/or unenforceable section would be lawful or enforceable if part of it were deleted, that part will be deemed to be deleted, and the rest of the section will continue in effect.

Law and jurisdiction

This disclaimer will be governed by and construed in accordance with Swiss law, and any disputes relating to this disclaimer will be subject to the exclusive jurisdiction of the courts of Switzerland.